HIIT It HARD!

Beginner's Guide to Weight Loss and Body Sculpting

by Bruce Goldwell

Copyright © 2023 Bruce Goldwell

All rights reserved

Disclaimer:

The information provided in this book is intended for general informational purposes only and is not a substitute for professional advice, diagnosis, or treatment. Always seek the advice of your physician or other qualified health provider with any questions you may have regarding a medical condition, diet, fitness, or any other health-related program. Never disregard professional medical advice or delay in seeking it because of something you have read in this book.

The author and publisher are not responsible for any specific health or allergy needs that may require medical supervision and are not liable for any damages or negative consequences from any treatment, action, application, or preparation, to any person reading or following the information in this book. Reliance on any information provided by this book is solely at your own risk.

Before starting any health or fitness program, it is recommended to consult with a qualified healthcare professional, fitness trainer, or nutritionist to ensure that the chosen activities or dietary plans are suitable for your individual needs and health status.

Remember, the results of any health or fitness program may vary from person to person. Consistency, dedication, and a personalized approach are crucial factors in achieving your health and fitness goals.

Always use your best judgment and consult with professionals when making decisions about your health.

DO YOU SUPPORT VETERANS?

Your _feedback_ is invaluable in improving my authorship.

As a proud Vietnam Veteran, I dedicate my life to supporting fellow Veterans in need.

**I humbly ask for your assistance.**

You can make a difference in the lives of vets as well as my own by simply **_"reading and reviewing"_** my books, before sharing them with your family and friends.

With your help, I can expand the reach of my novels and grow my community of readers. As the fan base strengthens, so will my book royalties, **_allowing me to not only channel financial aid towards homeless veterans_**, but also extend support to anyone facing life's challenges.

"Your Review holds immense power";

together, we can change lives.

Visit www.imalocalauthor.com for info on my books.

Bruce Goldwell

Table of Contents

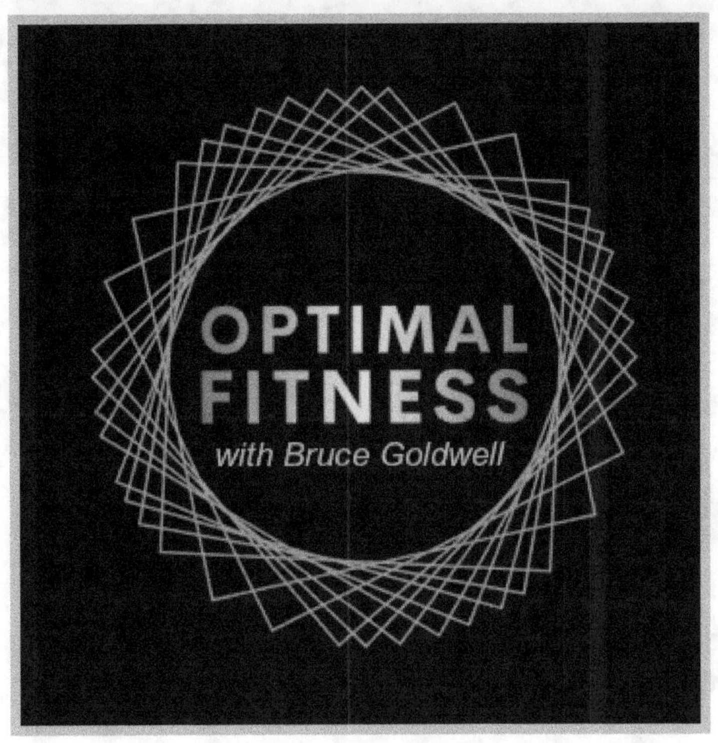

HIIT It HARD!

Beginner's Guide to Weight Loss and Body Sculpting

"Wisdom isn't knowing everything-

it's knowing when to learn from others."

Revolutionizing Fitness

The Rise and Power of High-Intensity Interval Training (HIIT)

High-Intensity Interval Training (HIIT) has emerged as a dynamic and transformative approach to cardiovascular exercise, captivating fitness enthusiasts with its unique blend of intensity and efficiency. This training method involves alternating short bursts of vigorous, anaerobic exercise with brief periods of rest or lower-intensity activity. Championed by registered dietitians like Cynthia Sass, HIIT has risen to prominence due to its time efficiency and a myriad of potential health benefits.

The structure of HIIT workouts is characterized by powerful, high-intensity exercises such as sprints or burpees, interspersed with intervals of rest or lower-intensity activity. This deliberate alternation allows individuals to attain substantial cardiovascular and metabolic advantages in a fraction of the time required for traditional steady-state cardio exercises.

In this exploration of HIIT, we delve into the multifaceted benefits that extend beyond conventional workout routines. From the enhancement of cardiovascular health to the preservation of muscle mass, HIIT has redefined the landscape of fitness. Its efficiency is underscored by the phenomenon of excess post-exercise oxygen consumption (EPOC), leading to sustained calorie burning even after the workout concludes.

This comprehensive overview will not only shed light on the physiological advantages of HIIT, including increased metabolic rate, fat loss, and improved oxygen consumption but will also navigate through various types of HIIT workouts, offering versatility to individuals based on their fitness levels and goals.

However, while the benefits of HIIT are compelling, safety considerations are paramount. Particularly for newcomers to exercise or those with underlying health conditions, a cautious approach is advised. Consulting with healthcare professionals before embarking on a HIIT program, especially concerning cardiovascular health, is a prudent step. The importance of proper warm-up and cool-down periods cannot be overstated, serving as crucial elements to mitigate the risk of injury and allow the body to adapt to the intensity of HIIT exercises.

In conclusion, the surge in popularity of High-Intensity Interval Training is not merely a fitness trend but a paradigm shift in achieving optimal health through effective and efficient cardiovascular exercise. With authoritative references from institutions such as the American College of Sports Medicine, PubMed Central, and Harvard Health Publishing, this exploration aims to provide a well-rounded understanding of HIIT, empowering individuals to make informed choices on their journey to fitness and well-being.

High-Intensity Interval Training (HIIT)

High-Intensity Interval Training (HIIT) is a form of cardiovascular exercise that alternates between short bursts of intense anaerobic exercise and less intense recovery periods. This type of training has gained popularity due to its time efficiency and potential health benefits. HIIT workouts typically involve short bursts of high-intensity exercises, such as sprints or burpees, followed by brief periods of rest or lower-intensity exercise. The structure of HIIT allows individuals to achieve significant cardiovascular and metabolic benefits in a shorter amount of time compared to traditional steady-state cardio exercises.

Benefits of HIIT

1. Improved Cardiovascular Health: HIIT has been shown to improve cardiovascular health by increasing the heart's ability to pump blood more efficiently and improving overall circulation. The intense intervals push the heart to work harder, leading to improved cardiovascular function over time.

2. Increased Metabolic Rate: HIIT can boost metabolism and increase the body's calorie-burning potential even after the workout is completed. This phenomenon, known as excess post-exercise oxygen consumption (EPOC),

results in continued calorie burning for hours after the workout.

3. Time Efficiency: One of the primary advantages of HIIT is its time efficiency. With shorter workout durations, individuals can achieve similar or even greater benefits compared to longer, steady-state cardio sessions.

4. Fat Loss: HIIT has been associated with fat loss, particularly abdominal fat. The combination of high-intensity intervals and EPOC can contribute to greater fat burning and improved body composition.

5. Muscle Retention: Unlike traditional steady-state cardio, which may lead to muscle loss over time, HIIT has been shown to help preserve muscle mass while promoting fat loss.

6. Improved Oxygen Consumption: HIIT can enhance the body's ability to consume oxygen during exercise, leading to improved endurance and overall fitness levels.

7. Regulated Blood Sugar Levels: Research suggests that HIIT may help regulate blood sugar levels and improve insulin sensitivity, making it beneficial for individuals with or at risk for type 2 diabetes.

Types of HIIT Workouts

There are various ways to structure a HIIT workout, and the specific exercises and intervals can be tailored to individual fitness levels and goals. Some common types of HIIT workouts include:

Tabata: Tabata training consists of 20 seconds of ultra-high-intensity exercise followed by 10 seconds of rest, repeated for a total of 8 rounds (4 minutes).

The Little Method: This method involves 60 seconds of intense exercise followed by 75 seconds of rest or low-intensity exercise, repeated for a total of 12 rounds (27 minutes).

10-20-30 Protocol: This protocol involves 30 seconds of low intensity, 20 seconds at a moderate intensity, and 10 seconds at high intensity, repeated for multiple cycles.

Customized Intervals: Individuals can also create their own customized intervals based on their fitness level and preferences.

Safety Considerations

While HIIT offers numerous benefits, it is essential to approach this form of training with caution, especially for individuals who are new to exercise or have underlying health conditions. It is advisable to consult with a healthcare professional before starting a HIIT program, particularly if there are concerns about cardiovascular health or other medical issues.

Additionally, proper warm-up and cool-down periods are crucial when engaging in HIIT workouts to reduce the risk of injury and allow the body to adapt to the intensity of the exercises.

In conclusion, High-Intensity Interval Training (HIIT) is an effective and efficient form of cardiovascular exercise that offers a wide range of health benefits, including improved cardiovascular health, increased metabolic rate, fat loss, muscle retention, improved oxygen consumption, and regulated blood sugar levels. With various types of workouts available and its time efficiency, HIIT has become a popular choice for individuals looking to maximize their workout results in a shorter amount of time.

Top 3 Authoritative Reference Publications or Domain Names Used to Define HIIT:

1. American College of Sports Medicine (ACSM): The ACSM is a widely recognized authority in sports medicine and exercise science, providing evidence-based guidelines and recommendations for physical activity and fitness.

2. PubMed Central: PubMed Central is a free digital archive of biomedical and life sciences journal literature, providing access to a vast collection of research articles related to exercise physiology and training methods.

3. Harvard Health Publishing: Harvard Health Publishing offers authoritative health information from the experts at Harvard Medical School, including articles on fitness, exercise physiology, and the benefits of different workout regimens.

Navigating the HIIT Terrain

Unraveling the Dynamics and Benefits

Embarking on the journey of High-Intensity Interval Training (HIIT) is not merely stepping onto the treadmill; it's a deliberate choice to redefine the way we approach cardiovascular exercise. In this chapter, we unravel the intricacies of HIIT, diving into a spectrum of questions that form the foundation of understanding this dynamic and transformative training method.

What is High-Intensity Interval Training (HIIT)?

High-Intensity Interval Training (HIIT) is a form of cardiovascular exercise that involves alternating short bursts of intense activity with equally short recovery periods. This type of workout is designed to improve overall fitness, increase muscle strength, and maximize caloric expenditure in a relatively short amount of time. HIIT workouts can be tailored to individual fitness levels and can be performed using various modes of exercises, such as running, cycling, swimming, or bodyweight exercises.

The main principle behind HIIT is the contrast between high-intensity intervals and low-intensity recovery periods. During the high-intensity phase, one would push their body to perform at its maximum capacity (typically reaching around 80-95% of their maximum heart rate). Following this, the lower intensity or active recovery period allows the heart rate and breathing to slow down before ramping up for the next high-intensity interval.

The advantages of HIIT include its efficiency in delivering significant improvements in cardiovascular health, muscular endurance, and fat burning within a compact training time. Moreover, it has been shown to boost metabolism due to its afterburn effect - a phenomenon wherein the body continues burning calories at an elevated rate post-workout. The easily customizable nature of HIIT workouts makes them appealing for individuals with varying fitness levels and goals.

In conclusion, High-Intensity Interval Training is a versatile and time-efficient workout method that combines intensive exercise bouts and recovery periods, offering numerous health benefits while challenging traditional workout patterns.

How does HIIT differ from traditional steady-state cardio?

High-intensity interval training (HIIT) differs from traditional steady-state cardio in several ways:

1. Intensity: HIIT involves alternating between short bursts of high-intensity exercise and lower intensity recovery periods. In contrast, steady-state cardio maintains a consistent intensity throughout the workout.

2. Duration: HIIT workouts are typically shorter in duration, lasting anywhere from 10-30 minutes. Steady-state cardio workouts can last longer, often ranging from 30-60 minutes or more.

3. Approach: HIIT focuses on pushing the body to its limits during high-intensity intervals to boost cardiovascular and metabolic health rapidly. Steady-state cardio emphasizes maintaining a sustainable pace for a prolonged period, promoting overall endurance and aerobic capacity.

4. Calorie Burn and Afterburn Effect: Due to its intensity, HIIT burns calories at a faster rate than traditional cardio and can result in a higher caloric burn overall due to the afterburn effect (EPOC), where the body continues to burn calories post-exercise. Steady-state cardio may burn fewer calories during the workout and have minimal afterburn effect.

5. Adaptability: HIIT workouts can be tailored to various fitness levels and exercise preferences by adjusting the length and intensity of intervals, making it accessible to a wide range of individuals. Steady-state cardio also allows for adaptability as one

What are the potential health benefits of HIIT?

As we venture into the physiological realm, we unravel the myriad of health benefits that HIIT promises. From enhancing cardiovascular health to elevating metabolic rates and promoting fat loss, HIIT emerges as a powerhouse in the world of fitness.

High Intensity Interval Training (HIIT) offers a variety of potential health benefits, including:

1. Improved cardiovascular health: HIIT has been shown to increase the efficiency of the heart and blood vessels, strengthening these vital components.

2. Enhanced metabolic rates: Through its high-intensity nature, HIIT boosts metabolism for a longer duration after the workout, leading to greater calorie expenditure.

3. Promoted fat loss: By encouraging fat oxidation and increased calorie burning, HIIT promotes overall fat loss.

4. Increased muscle strength and endurance: Incorporating resistance training in HIIT can lead to increased muscle strength.

5. Better blood sugar control: Studies have shown that HIIT can help lower blood sugar levels by increasing insulin sensitivity.

6. Reduced blood pressure: Regular HIIT workouts can lead to a reduction in both systolic and diastolic blood

pressure.

7. Improved mental well-being: The endorphin release from HIIT workouts aids in improving mood and reducing stress levels.

8. Time-efficient exercise: A significant benefit of HIIT is that it allows for an effective workout in less time when compared to moderate-intensity exercises.

These health benefits make HIIT an attractive option, particularly for those with busy schedules or looking for efficient workouts to maximize results.

How long should a typical HIIT workout last?

Time efficiency is a hallmark of HIIT. Here, we navigate the optimal duration for a HIIT session, demystifying how it compares to the time commitment required for traditional cardio workouts.

A typical High-Intensity Interval Training (HIIT) workout should last between 20 to 30 minutes. This time frame is considered optimal as it allows for an effective combination of intense, short bursts of activity, alternating with sufficient recovery periods. The short duration not only makes HIIT workouts more manageable and time-efficient but also enables one to maintain intensity throughout the session without losing effectiveness. Compared to traditional cardio workouts, which often require longer periods of sustained effort, HIIT offers similar or superior benefits within a shorter time span.

What types of exercises are suitable for HIIT?

Identifying high-intensity exercises that seamlessly integrate into a HIIT routine is crucial. Discover the range of exercises suited for HIIT and learn how to tailor them to your individual fitness levels and aspirations.

High-intensity exercises suitable for HIIT routines include:

1. Jump squats

2. Burpees

3. Mountain climbers

4. High knees

5. Box jumps

6. Jumping lunges

7. Sprints

8. Push-ups

9. Split squats

10. Tuck jumps

11. Plank jacks

12. Bicycle crunches

13. Speed skaters

14. Kettlebell swings

15. Battle ropes

To tailor these exercises to your individual fitness levels and aspirations, you can adjust the intensity, duration, and rest intervals between each exercise according to your capabilities and goals.

What is excess post-exercise ...

...oxygen consumption (EPOC) and how does it contribute to calorie burning?

Excess post-exercise oxygen consumption (EPOC) is a physiological process that occurs after intense physical activity, where the body's oxygen consumption remains elevated for a period of time, usually several hours or up to 48 hours. This increased oxygen intake helps to restore the body back to its pre-exercise state and promotes various processes such as removing lactate, replenishing energy stores, and repairing damaged tissues.

EPOC contributes to calorie burning because the body requires additional energy during this recovery period. The increased metabolic rate from EPOC further boosts calorie expenditure even after the workout session has ended. This is particularly evident in high-intensity interval training (HIIT), where short bursts of intense exercise followed by brief recovery periods maximize EPOC effects.

The science behind EPOC revolves around the body's need to recover from a stressed state brought on by intense exercise. HIIT workouts provide a significant stimulus that elevates heart rate and activates various muscle fibers, leading to increased oxygen demand during exercise as well as post-exercise recovery. Oxygen plays a crucial role in metabolic processes that produce energy for the body through cellular respiration, which makes it necessary for sustaining numerous physiological functions.

During EPOC, calorie burning is extended because of the heightened metabolic rate and increased utilization of fat stores. Lipolysis, which is the breakdown of fats into fatty acids and glycerol, is enhanced during this period due to higher levels of circulating hormones such as adrenaline and noradrenaline, which promote fat oxidation. Thus, in addition to burning calories during exercise, there is a continuation of calorie expenditure even after an intense HIIT workout session.

In conclusion, excess post-exercise oxygen consumption (EPOC) is a phenomenon that contributes significantly to calorie burning after strenuous physical activity. It provides a rationale for incorporating high-intensity interval training (HIIT) in one's workout routine for maximizing calorie-burning benefits, as EPOC extends the energy expenditure beyond the exercise session itself.

Can HIIT help with muscle retention?

High-Intensity Interval Training (HIIT) has gained popularity as an effective way to simultaneously improve cardiovascular fitness and muscle retention. Unlike steady-state cardio, which tends to focus solely on improving cardiovascular endurance, HIIT uniquely impacts muscle mass due to the high-intensity nature of the exercises involved.

The core principle of HIIT is alternating between short bursts of intense exercise and periods of active recovery or rest. This leads to two primary factors that differentiate HIIT from steady-state cardio in terms of muscle preservation:

1. Anaerobic Nature of HIIT: The high-intensity intervals in a HIIT workout tax the anaerobic energy system, which relies on energy stored in muscles for quick bursts of power. As a result, HIIT stimulates muscle fibers more effectively than steady-state cardio, thus supporting the preservation -- and even growth -- of muscle mass.

2. Excess Post-Exercise Oxygen Consumption (EPOC): HIIT increases your metabolic rate for hours after a workout, known as the afterburn effect, or EPOC. This effect not only aids fat-burning but also stimulates muscle protein synthesis (MPS), helping retain and rebuild muscle tissue.

These factors contribute to a unique impact that supports both muscular development and cardiovascular fitness simultaneously. Therefore, while steady-state cardio may not have a significant impact on muscle retention or growth, HIIT offers the potential to preserve and enhance muscle mass while still improving overall endurance and fitness levels.

Are there different types of HIIT workouts?

High-Intensity Interval Training (HIIT) thrives on versatility, offering a spectrum of workout protocols that cater to different preferences, fitness levels, and goals. It's a departure from the one-size-fits-all approach, encouraging individuals to explore various HIIT workout methods. Here, we delve into some popular HIIT protocols, each bringing its own flavor to the dynamic world of interval training.

1. Tabata Training:

Tabata is a well-known and efficient HIIT protocol characterized by short, intense bursts of exercise followed by brief periods of rest. The classic Tabata structure involves 20 seconds of ultra-high-intensity exercise followed by 10 seconds of rest, repeated for a total of 8 rounds, resulting in a four-minute workout. This method is celebrated for its time efficiency and effectiveness in improving both aerobic and anaerobic fitness.

2. The Little Method:

The Little Method takes a slightly longer approach, with 60 seconds of intense exercise followed by 75 seconds of rest or low-intensity exercise. This sequence is repeated for a total of 12 rounds, culminating in a 27-minute workout. The Little Method offers a balance between intensity and duration, making it suitable for individuals who prefer a bit more extended HIIT session.

3. 10-20-30 Protocol:

This protocol introduces variability in intensity within each interval. It involves 30 seconds of low-intensity exercise, followed by 20 seconds at a moderate intensity, and concluding with 10 seconds of high-intensity effort. This cycle is then repeated for multiple rounds, allowing for a dynamic and varied workout experience. The 10-20-30 Protocol offers a blend of intensity levels, making it adaptable to different fitness levels and preferences.

4. Customized Intervals:

One of the beauties of HIIT is its adaptability. Individuals can create their own customized intervals based on their fitness levels, preferences, and specific goals. This flexibility allows for endless variations, incorporating a mix of cardio and strength exercises to create a personalized and effective HIIT routine.

5. Cardio and Strength Hybrid HIIT:

Some HIIT workouts integrate both cardiovascular and strength-training elements. This hybrid approach combines intense cardio intervals with bodyweight exercises or resistance training. Incorporating strength elements into HIIT adds a dimension of full-body conditioning, promoting muscle development alongside cardiovascular fitness.

6. Sports-Specific HIIT:

Tailoring HIIT to mimic the demands of specific sports is another approach. Athletes can design HIIT workouts that mirror the intensity and movement patterns of their chosen sport, contributing to sport-specific conditioning and performance enhancement.

By familiarizing yourself with these various HIIT protocols, you gain the tools to diversify your training routine and keep your workouts engaging and effective. The key lies in experimenting with different methods, discovering what resonates with your fitness goals, and enjoying the adaptability that HIIT brings to your exercise regimen. Whether you prefer the quick intensity of Tabata or the longer duration of The Little Method, the world of HIIT is rich with options to cater to your unique preferences and aspirations.

Is HIIT suitable for everyone, or are there safety considerations?

High-Intensity Interval Training (HIIT) stands as a dynamic and efficient fitness approach, yet its suitability for individuals varies based on factors such as fitness levels, health conditions, and prior exercise experience. As we explore the expansive benefits of HIIT, it's crucial to underscore the importance of safety considerations and tailor this high-intensity regimen to individual needs.

1. Individual Fitness Levels:

The adaptability of HIIT is a double-edged sword. While it can be customized to various fitness levels, the high-intensity nature of the workouts may pose challenges for beginners or those unaccustomed to rigorous exercise. Individuals with sedentary lifestyles or limited fitness experience might find it beneficial to gradually incorporate lower-intensity intervals before progressing to more intense HIIT sessions.

2. Underlying Health Conditions:

Safety concerns are particularly pertinent for individuals with pre-existing health conditions. Conditions such as cardiovascular issues, joint problems, or chronic illnesses may require a cautious approach. Consulting with healthcare professionals, including physicians and specialists, becomes imperative to ensure that HIIT aligns with individual health circumstances.

3. Potential Risks for Novices:

For newcomers to exercise, diving headfirst into high-intensity workouts can pose risks. Inadequate preparation and form can lead to injuries, especially in weight-bearing exercises. It's essential to emphasize the importance of proper guidance, including supervised workouts or training sessions led by qualified fitness instructors, to mitigate the risk of injuries for novices.

4. Impact on Joint Health:

The intensity of some HIIT exercises, particularly those involving jumping or high-impact movements, may exert stress on joints. Individuals with joint issues or arthritis may need modifications or alternative exercises to safeguard joint health. Low-impact variations can be incorporated to minimize stress on the joints while still reaping the benefits of HIIT.

5. Importance of Professional Guidance:

HIIT's effectiveness is maximized when coupled with proper form and technique. Enlisting the guidance of certified fitness professionals ensures that individuals perform exercises correctly, reducing the risk of injury. Professionals can also tailor HIIT workouts to accommodate individual fitness levels and goals, ensuring a safe and effective training experience.

6. Gradual Progression:

Safety considerations dictate a gradual approach to HIIT, especially for those new to high-intensity exercise. Slowly increasing the intensity and duration of workouts allows the body to adapt, reducing the likelihood of overexertion, burnout, or injury.

7. Monitoring Intensity and Recovery:

HIIT is characterized by a delicate balance of intense exercise and recovery periods. Striking the right balance is crucial for preventing overtraining and promoting adequate recovery. Monitoring individual energy levels, fatigue, and overall well-being is essential to tailor HIIT workouts effectively.

In conclusion, while HIIT offers a wealth of benefits, safety considerations are paramount. The suitability of HIIT for everyone hinges on an individual's fitness level, health status, and exercise history. By prioritizing safety, consulting healthcare professionals, and seeking guidance from qualified fitness professionals, individuals can unlock the transformative potential of HIIT while minimizing potential risks. This approach ensures a safe, effective, and sustainable fitness journey for individuals of diverse backgrounds and fitness levels.

What role does warm-up and cool-down play in HIIT?

Warm-Up: Preparing the Body for Intensity

The warm-up phase in High-Intensity Interval Training (HIIT) is a critical element that serves as a bridge between a sedentary state and the heightened intensity of the workout ahead. Recognizing the significance of a proper warm-up routine is essential for priming the body, mentally preparing for exertion, and mitigating the risk of injuries. Here's an exploration of the role warm-up plays in the context of HIIT:

1. Increased Blood Flow and Oxygen Delivery:

A well-structured warm-up involves low-intensity aerobic activities, such as brisk walking or light jogging, which gradually increase the heart rate and stimulate blood flow. This process enhances the delivery of oxygen to muscles, preparing them for the upcoming surge in demand during high-intensity intervals.

2. Improved Flexibility and Joint Mobility:

Dynamic stretching incorporated into the warm-up routine helps improve flexibility and joint mobility. This is particularly crucial in HIIT, where explosive and varied movements are common. Enhanced flexibility contributes to better range of motion, reducing the risk of strains or muscle pulls during the intense phases of the workout.

3. Mental Preparedness:

The warm-up phase is not just about physical preparation; it plays a vital role in mentally gearing up for the challenges of HIIT. As individuals engage in low-intensity exercises, they mentally transition from a state of rest to a heightened awareness of the upcoming intensity. This mental preparedness is integral to maintaining focus and maximizing effort during the high-intensity intervals.

4. Activation of Muscles:

Specific activation exercises targeting major muscle groups are often included in the warm-up. This activation primes the muscles for more explosive and powerful movements, reducing the risk of injury. It also helps individuals establish a mind-body connection, ensuring that the correct muscle groups are engaged during the subsequent high-intensity efforts.

Cool-Down: Easing the Body Out of Intensity

Just as the warm-up is crucial for transitioning into the intensity of HIIT, the cool-down phase is indispensable for transitioning out of it. The cool-down routine allows the body to gradually return to a state of rest and aids in the recovery process. Here's an exploration of the role cool-down plays in the context of HIIT:

1. Gradual Reduction of Heart Rate:

Engaging in low-intensity exercises during the cool-down, such as walking or gentle jogging, helps gradually lower the heart rate. This controlled reduction in heart rate allows the cardiovascular system to adjust more smoothly to the change in intensity, preventing abrupt fluctuations that may stress the heart.

2. Removal of Metabolic Byproducts:

Intense exercise produces metabolic byproducts, such as lactic acid, that can accumulate in muscles. The cool-down phase, which involves low-intensity movements, facilitates the removal of these byproducts by promoting blood circulation. This process contributes to faster recovery and minimizes muscle soreness.

3. Flexibility and Muscle Relaxation:

Incorporating static stretching during the cool-down helps to maintain and improve flexibility. Stretching the muscles when they are warm and pliable aids in preventing stiffness and promotes muscle relaxation, fostering a sense of physical well-being.

4. Enhanced Recovery:

The cool-down phase plays a crucial role in the overall recovery process. It allows the body to gradually transition from a state of heightened activity to a state of rest, reducing the risk of dizziness or light-headedness. It also supports the return of the respiratory and circulatory systems to baseline levels.

In conclusion, both the warm-up and cool-down phases are integral components of a well-rounded HIIT workout. They contribute to injury prevention, improve performance, and support the body in adapting to the intensity of the exercise. Incorporating these elements into a HIIT routine enhances the overall effectiveness of the workout and promotes a safer and more sustainable fitness experience.

How can individuals tailor HIIT to their fitness levels and goals?

Customizing High-Intensity Interval Training (HIIT) allows individuals to optimize their workouts based on their unique fitness levels, preferences, and health goals. By tailoring HIIT, individuals can strike a balance between pushing their limits and ensuring a safe and enjoyable exercise experience. Here's a comprehensive exploration of how individuals can personalize HIIT to align with their individual needs:

1. Assessing Fitness Levels:

Understanding your current fitness level is the first step in tailoring HIIT. Novices may start with shorter sessions and lower-intensity intervals, gradually progressing as their endurance and strength improve. Experienced individuals can incorporate more challenging exercises and longer intervals, pushing their boundaries within safe limits.

2. Modifying Intensity and Duration:

HIIT's flexibility lies in its adjustable intensity and duration. Beginners can start with lower-intensity intervals, allowing for longer recovery periods. As fitness levels advance, individuals can progressively increase the intensity and reduce recovery times. Customizing the duration of both high-intensity and rest intervals is key to meeting specific fitness goals.

3. Choosing Appropriate Exercises:

The choice of exercises plays a pivotal role in tailoring HIIT. Individuals can select exercises that align with their fitness levels and preferences. Low-impact options, such as cycling or swimming, may be suitable for those with joint concerns, while more dynamic, high-impact exercises like burpees or jumping jacks may be chosen by those seeking a more intense challenge.

4. Incorporating Strength Training:

HIIT can be customized to include strength training elements, providing a holistic workout experience. Integrating bodyweight exercises, resistance training, or incorporating weights can enhance muscle development alongside cardiovascular benefits. This customization allows individuals to target specific muscle groups or overall body conditioning based on their goals.

5. Adapting for Health Considerations:

Individuals with specific health considerations can tailor HIIT to accommodate their needs. For those with cardiovascular issues, low-impact exercises or modified intervals may be preferred. Individuals with joint concerns can opt for exercises that minimize impact, while those with metabolic goals may focus on optimizing fat-burning intervals.

6. Varied Protocols for Diversification:

HIIT comes in various protocols, each offering a unique approach to interval training. Individuals can experiment with protocols like Tabata, The Little Method, or create their own customized intervals. Diversifying protocols keeps workouts engaging and targets different aspects of fitness, allowing for a well-rounded approach.

7. Setting Specific Goals:

Tailoring HIIT involves aligning workouts with specific health and wellness goals. Whether the aim is fat loss, cardiovascular improvement, or muscle development, customization allows individuals to structure HIIT to meet these objectives. Setting realistic and measurable goals helps guide the customization process.

8. Listening to the Body:

Customization involves a continuous dialogue with the body. Listening to how the body responds to different exercises and intensity levels is crucial. This intuitive approach allows individuals to adjust their workouts in real-time, ensuring a balance between pushing limits and avoiding overexertion or injury.

9. Consistency and Progression:

Customizing HIIT is an ongoing process that involves consistency and progression. Regularly reassessing fitness levels, adjusting intervals, and incorporating new exercises contribute to sustained progress. Gradual progression prevents plateaus and ensures that workouts remain challenging and effective.

10. Seeking Professional Guidance:

Consulting with fitness professionals or personal trainers can provide valuable insights into tailoring HIIT effectively. Professionals can assess individual fitness levels, offer personalized advice, and create customized workout plans that align with specific goals while ensuring safety and efficacy.

In conclusion, unlocking the secrets of customization in HIIT empowers individuals to shape their fitness journey according to their unique needs and aspirations. By assessing fitness levels, modifying intensity and duration, choosing appropriate exercises, and considering health considerations, individuals can craft HIIT workouts that are not only effective but also enjoyable and sustainable over the long term.

Navigating the Scientific Landscape of HIIT

Insights from Authoritative Sources

Embarking on a journey of High-Intensity Interval Training (HIIT) goes beyond the sweat-inducing workouts; it delves into the realm of evidence-based research. The chapter that follows serves as your compass, guiding you through the intricate landscape of HIIT by unraveling the latest findings from esteemed sources like the American College of Sports Medicine (ACSM), PubMed Central, and Harvard Health Publishing. Here's a comprehensive exploration of what the research from these authoritative sources reveals about HIIT:

1. American College of Sports Medicine (ACSM):

The ACSM stands as a beacon in the field of sports medicine and exercise science, providing evidence-based guidelines and recommendations for physical activity and fitness. Research from the ACSM underscores the efficacy of HIIT in improving cardiovascular health, enhancing metabolic function, and promoting overall fitness. The organization's findings delve into the nuanced aspects of HIIT, offering insights into optimal protocols, safety considerations, and the adaptability of HIIT for diverse populations.

2. PubMed Central:

As a free digital archive of biomedical and life sciences journal literature, PubMed Central houses a wealth of research articles related to exercise physiology and training methods. Research from PubMed Central enriches our understanding of the physiological responses triggered by HIIT, including its impact on oxygen consumption, fat metabolism, and muscle retention. These findings provide a scientific foundation for tailoring HIIT to individual goals and optimizing its effectiveness.

3. Harvard Health Publishing:

Harvard Health Publishing, with its commitment to disseminating authoritative health information, contributes valuable insights into the benefits and considerations of HIIT. Research from Harvard Health Publishing delves into the broader implications of HIIT on overall well-being, addressing topics such as its role in regulating blood sugar levels, its potential impact on chronic diseases, and its relevance for diverse age groups. This research aids in painting a holistic picture of HIIT's multifaceted benefits.

4. Cardiovascular Health:

Authoritative research consistently highlights HIIT's profound impact on cardiovascular health. Studies from ACSM emphasize how the alternating cycles of intense exercise and rest periods lead to improved heart function, enhanced circulation, and increased efficiency in pumping blood. This not only contributes to cardiovascular endurance but also has implications for reducing the risk of heart-related issues.

5. Metabolic Rate and Fat Loss:

HIIT's ability to elevate metabolic rate and promote fat loss is a recurrent theme in research. PubMed Central findings shed light on the mechanisms behind the "afterburn" effect, scientifically known as excess post-exercise oxygen consumption (EPOC). This extended calorie-burning phase post-HIIT is explored, offering insights into how HIIT contributes to sustainable weight management.

6. Adaptability for Diverse Goals:

The research landscape, as curated by these authoritative sources, underscores HIIT's adaptability for diverse fitness goals. Whether individuals aim for weight loss, muscle development, or overall fitness improvement, the customization potential of HIIT is substantiated. This adaptability makes HIIT a versatile and accessible option for individuals with varying aspirations.

7. Safety Considerations and Guidelines:

ACSM research provides essential safety considerations and guidelines for implementing HIIT effectively. From recommendations for proper warm-up and cool-down routines to insights into gradual progression, the research offers a roadmap for individuals to navigate HIIT safely. This evidence-based approach ensures that the benefits of HIIT are harnessed without compromising individual well-being.

8. Role in Chronic Disease Management:

Harvard Health Publishing explores HIIT's potential role in managing chronic diseases, such as type 2 diabetes. Research indicates that HIIT may positively influence insulin sensitivity and blood sugar regulation. This information becomes a cornerstone for individuals seeking holistic health improvements beyond just fitness.

In conclusion, the amalgamation of research findings from authoritative sources provides health-conscious individuals with a robust foundation for understanding HIIT. The insights gleaned from ACSM, PubMed Central, and Harvard Health Publishing collectively form a compass, guiding individuals through the nuanced landscape of HIIT. Armed with evidence-based knowledge, health-conscious individuals are empowered to optimize their fitness journey, ensuring not only effectiveness but also safety and longevity in their pursuit of health and well-being.

Fueling Your HIIT Journey

A Comprehensive Guide to Nutrition for Optimal Performance and Results

Nutrition plays a crucial role in supporting High-Intensity Interval Training (HIIT) and optimizing performance, recovery, and overall fitness outcomes. Consider the following nutritional considerations when engaging in HIIT:

1. Pre-Workout Nutrition:

- Timing: Consume a balanced meal 2-3 hours before your HIIT session to provide a source of energy.

- Carbohydrates: Include complex carbohydrates like whole grains, fruits, and vegetables for sustained energy.

- Protein: Include a moderate amount of protein to support muscle function.

2. Hydration:

- Pre-Workout: Ensure you are well-hydrated before starting your HIIT session.

- During Workout: Sip water during your workout, especially if it's an extended session.

- Post-Workout: Rehydrate with water or a sports drink containing electrolytes if the workout was particularly intense and you sweated heavily.

3. Post-Workout Nutrition:

- Timing: Consume a post-workout meal or snack within 30 minutes to an hour after exercising.

- Protein: Prioritize protein intake to support muscle repair and growth.

- Carbohydrates: Include carbohydrates to replenish glycogen stores depleted during the workout.

- Hydration: Continue to hydrate to replace fluids lost through sweat.

4. Macronutrient Balance:

- Carbohydrates: They are a primary energy source for HIIT. Include both complex and simple carbohydrates in your diet.

- Protein: Essential for muscle repair and recovery. Include lean protein sources like poultry, fish, tofu, or legumes.

- Fats: Healthy fats provide a source of sustained energy. Include sources like avocados, nuts, and olive oil.

5. Individualized Nutrition:

- Consider individual factors such as age, gender, weight, and specific fitness goals when planning your nutrition around HIIT.

- If you have any pre-existing medical conditions or dietary restrictions, consult with a healthcare professional or a registered dietitian for personalized advice.

6. Supplements:

- While a well-balanced diet should ideally provide all the nutrients you need, some individuals may benefit from supplements.

- Common supplements for those engaged in HIIT may include protein powder for convenient post-workout protein intake, and electrolyte supplements if you sweat heavily during workouts.

7. Experiment and Listen to Your Body:

- Everyone's nutritional needs can vary. Experiment with different pre- and post-workout meals to see what works best for you.

- Pay attention to how your body responds to different foods and adjust your nutrition accordingly.

8. Consider Goals:

   - Tailor your nutrition to align with your specific fitness goals. For example, if your goal is fat loss, you may focus on creating a calorie deficit, while those aiming for muscle gain may need a calorie surplus and higher protein intake.

9. Avoid Heavy Meals Before HIIT:

   - Consuming a heavy meal immediately before HIIT can lead to discomfort. Opt for a lighter snack if you're working out shortly after a meal.

Heavy metals are toxic elements that can be harmful to the human body when ingested in excessive amounts over time. Common heavy metals that individuals should avoid or minimize in their diet include:

Lead: Found in contaminated water, certain canned goods, and some traditional medicines.

Mercury: Found in certain types of fish, especially large predatory fish like shark, swordfish, king mackerel, and tile-fish.

Arsenic: Found in rice, certain types of seafood, and

contaminated water.

Cadmium: Present in some shellfish, kidney, and liver.

To minimize exposure to heavy metals, individuals should aim for a varied and balanced diet, choose a variety of fish low in mercury, source grains carefully, and be mindful of potential contaminants in water sources.

While the recommendation to avoid heavy meals before HIIT is primarily related to the composition and size of the meal, it is also in line with promoting overall digestive comfort during intense physical activity. Opting for a lighter snack ensures that the body has enough energy without overloading the digestive system, allowing individuals to perform their best during HIIT without experiencing discomfort.

10. Long-Term Nutrition:

- Consistency in maintaining a well-balanced diet over the long term is key for sustained energy levels, recovery, and overall health.

Always remember that individual nutritional needs can vary, and it's essential to find an approach that works best for your body and aligns with your specific health and fitness goals. If you have any concerns or specific dietary needs, consulting with a registered dietitian or nutrition professional is recommended.

Unleashing the Power of Home Fitness with HIIT

In the dynamic landscape of fitness, the concept of High-Intensity Interval Training (HIIT) has emerged as a revolutionary game-changer, offering a potent fusion of effectiveness and efficiency. What makes HIIT truly transformative is its adaptability, breaking free from the constraints of traditional workout settings and finding its stride in the comfort of your own home.

No longer confined to the walls of a gym or the restrictions of specialized equipment, HIIT has opened the door to a new era of accessible and impactful fitness. This approach to exercise revolves around short bursts of intense activity interspersed with brief periods of rest or lower-intensity exercises. The beauty of HIIT lies not only in its ability to torch calories and elevate fitness levels but also in its versatility and convenience, making it an ideal candidate for home workouts.

This introduction marks the beginning of a journey into the world of at-home HIIT, where the living room transforms into a dynamic fitness arena and everyday household items become the tools for transformative workouts. Explore the flexibility and simplicity of integrating HIIT into your home routine, unlocking a pathway to improved cardiovascular health, enhanced metabolism, and a body that thrives on the intensity of efficient, home-based workouts.

Join us as we delve into the strategies, exercises, and motivational insights that make at-home HIIT not just a possibility but a compelling choice for individuals seeking a convenient and impactful approach to fitness. Whether you're a fitness enthusiast looking to diversify your routine or a beginner seeking an accessible entry point into the world of high-intensity training, this exploration of at-home HIIT is your guide to realizing the full potential of fitness within the familiar confines of home. Get ready to redefine your understanding of home workouts as we embark on a journey where every living space becomes a canvas for sculpting a healthier, stronger, and more vibrant you.

Performing High-Intensity Interval Training (HIIT) at home can be both effective and convenient. Here are some essential things you'll need to get started with HIIT at home:

1. Space:

   - Ensure you have a designated workout space with enough room to move freely. Clear away any obstacles or potential hazards to create a safe environment.

2. Comfortable Workout Attire:

   - Wear comfortable athletic clothing and supportive shoes to facilitate movement and prevent injuries.

3. Interval Timer or Stopwatch:

   - An interval timer or a stopwatch is crucial for timing your high-intensity and rest intervals during the workout. Many workout apps and online timers are available to guide you through HIIT sessions.

4. Exercise Mat:

- comfortable exercise mat provides a cushioned surface for floor exercises and adds support to your joints.

5. Water Bottle:

- Staying hydrated is essential during any workout. Have a water bottle within reach to stay fueled and replenish fluids as needed.

6. Smartphone or Tablet:

- Many HIIT workouts can be guided through fitness apps or online videos. Ensure you have a device with a reliable internet connection to access workouts.

7. HIIT Workouts or Programs:

- Collect a variety of HIIT workouts or follow specific programs tailored to your fitness level. You can find workouts on fitness apps, YouTube, or through specialized fitness programs.

Best HIIT Workout DVDs on Amazon

https://amzn.to/417ZtQZ

8. Chair or Bench:

- Some HIIT exercises may involve step-ups, tricep dips, or other moves that utilize a stable surface. A sturdy chair or bench can serve this purpose.

9. Resistance Bands:

- Resistance bands add an extra challenge to

bodyweight exercises and can be easily incorporated into HIIT workouts to target various muscle groups.

10. Dumbbells or Kettlebells:

- Adding weights to your HIIT routine can increase the intensity and help build strength. Start with a moderate weight that challenges you but allows for proper form.

11. Mirror:

- Having a mirror in your workout space allows you to check and maintain proper form during exercises, reducing the risk of injury.

12. Motivational Music:

- Create a playlist of your favorite energetic tunes to keep you motivated and enhance the overall enjoyment of your workout. If working with an HIIT DVD, music is of course provided in the workout video. For runners and other outdoor activities, music for HIIT workouts is available on Amazon:

13. Fitness Tracker or Heart Rate Monitor:

- Monitoring your heart rate and tracking your progress can provide valuable insights into your fitness level and help you tailor your workouts.

Remember to start at your fitness level and gradually increase the intensity as you become more comfortable with the exercises. Consult with a healthcare professional before beginning any new exercise program, especially if you have existing health concerns.

For Body Building

Vince Sant is a fitness entrepreneur, personal trainer, and co-founder of the fitness brand V Shred. V Shred is known for its online fitness programs, workout plans, and nutritional guidance. Vince Sant, along with his brother Nick, established V Shred to make fitness and nutrition accessible to a wide audience through digital platforms.

Vince has gained popularity through his presence on social media and YouTube, where he shares workout routines, fitness tips, and nutritional advice. He is known for his expertise in creating effective and diverse workout programs that cater to various fitness levels and goals.

Vince emphasizes the importance of proper form and technique when lifting weights for High-Intensity Interval Training (HIIT). While specific recommendations may evolve, the general principles are likely to remain consistent. Here are some common guidelines that fitness experts, including Vince Sant, often advocate:

1. Focus on Form:

- Emphasize proper form over lifting heavy weights. Maintaining correct form reduces the risk of injury and ensures that you're targeting the intended muscle groups effectively.

2. Start with Warm-Up:

- Begin each HIIT session with a proper warm-up. This helps prepare your muscles for the upcoming intensity and reduces the risk of strains or injuries.

3. Incorporate Compound Movements:

- Include compound exercises that engage multiple muscle groups simultaneously. Compound movements are efficient for burning calories and building strength in a time-efficient manner, which aligns with the principles of HIIT.

4. Utilize Full Range of Motion:

- Perform exercises through their full range of motion to maximize muscle engagement and flexibility. This contributes to the overall effectiveness of the workout.

5. Controlled Movements:

- Maintain control throughout each movement. Avoid

using momentum to lift weights, as controlled
movements enhance muscle activation and reduce the
risk of injury.

6. Progress Gradually:

- Gradually increase the intensity and weight of your
workouts. Progressive overload is key for continued
improvement, but it's important to progress at a pace
that allows your muscles and joints to adapt.

7. Include Variability:

- Incorporate a variety of exercises to target different
muscle groups and keep your workouts dynamic. This
helps prevent plateaus and keeps the workouts
challenging.

8. Listen to Your Body:

- Pay attention to your body's signals. If you
experience pain (not to be confused with the normal
discomfort of a challenging workout), it's crucial to
modify or stop the exercise to prevent injury.

9. Combine with Cardio:

- Blend weightlifting with cardiovascular exercises to create a well-rounded HIIT routine. This combination enhances both strength and cardiovascular fitness.

10. Proper Breathing:

- Focus on proper breathing during exercises. Oxygenating your muscles is essential for endurance and overall workout performance.

Remember that these recommendations are general guidelines, and individual variations may apply. It's advisable to consult with a fitness professional or healthcare provider, especially if you have any existing health conditions or concerns. Additionally, for the most current advice from Vince Sant, checking his latest content or official platforms is recommended.

Do slow repetitions offer advantages for hypertrophy?

In hypertrophy-focused workouts, the emphasis lies in prolonging the time under tension to enhance endurance and promote muscle growth through the fatigue of muscle fibers. This typically involves executing a greater number of repetitions and deliberately slowing down the eccentric or lowering phase of the movement, commonly referred to as experiencing the burn.

Understanding Eccentric, Concentric, and Isometric Phases in Exercise Movements

These three terms delineate distinct phases within a movement and illuminate how your muscles respond during each stage.

In the **eccentric phase**, your muscles undergo lengthening as they encounter a resistance greater than the force they produce. Visualize this as the lowering phase, such as descending into a squat, lowering during a pull-up, or lowering your arm in a bicep curl.

Conversely, the **isometric phase** denotes a motionless segment of the exercise. This might involve a pause at the apex of a pull-up or a still moment at the nadir of a push-up or squat. Phrases like **"isometric hold"** or **"isometric pulse"** signify maintaining a position or executing small pulsing movements, as commonly seen in Pilates routines.

In the concentric phase, muscle tension intensifies, causing muscle fibers to contract or shorten as you exert force against a resistance. This phase typically represents the exertion of power, such as pulling yourself up in a pull-up, the upward motion of a push-up, or the ascent in a squat. Understanding and incorporating these phases into your workout routine can enhance your overall exercise effectiveness and target specific aspects of muscle engagement.

Research findings revealed that Super-Slow training led to approximately a 50% higher improvement ($p<0.001$) in strength for both males and females compared to conventional speed training. In Study 1, participants in the Super-Slow training group demonstrated an average increase of 12.0 kg, while the regular speed group exhibited an increase of 8.0 kg ($p<0.001$).

Suggestion:

Muscle growth occurs when you challenge your muscles beyond their usual limits, inducing slight damage that prompts the process of strain and repair. The type of muscle development—whether more bulk or a leaner, more defined appearance—depends on your approach to resistance training. Employing heavy weights with fewer repetitions fosters bulkier muscles, while lighter weights with higher repetitions promote firmer and more toned musculature. There's no secret formula; success hinges on the effort you invest. A balanced exercise regimen, encompassing aerobic, resistance, and varied resistance (weight-lifting) exercises with both high and low rep components, is integral for long-term benefits.

In the initial six months of a fitness program, a prudent strategy involves focusing on foundational exercises, such as three sets of 10 reps for each muscle group. This is because the distinctions between high and low repetition weight sets are marginal until an individual achieves significant strength, leanness, and muscular development. Prioritizing the establishment of a solid foundation is crucial before delving into intricate details—unless, of course, you specialize in power-lifting or aspire to a fitness model physique.

FIIT for Weight Loss

Unlocking the Potential of Functional Intensity Interval Training

Embark on a transformative journey towards weight loss through the dynamic realm of Functional Intensity Interval Training (FIIT). This chapter unravels the principles and benefits of FIIT, offering a comprehensive guide to harnessing its potential for achieving and sustaining weight loss goals.

Key Concepts:

1. Understanding FIIT:

- FIIT combines functional movements with high-intensity intervals, creating a workout approach that not only burns calories during the session but also enhances overall functional fitness. Delve into the fundamental concepts that distinguish FIIT from traditional exercise routines.

2. Metabolic Boost and Caloric Burn:

- Explore how FIIT's blend of functional movements and high-intensity intervals elevates your metabolic rate, fostering increased caloric burn both during and after workouts. Uncover the science behind FIIT's efficiency in torching calories, a vital component of successful weight loss.

3. Functional Movements for Full-Body Engagement:

   - FIIT emphasizes functional exercises that mimic real-life movements, engaging multiple muscle groups simultaneously. Learn how these compound movements not only contribute to calorie expenditure but also enhance overall strength, mobility, and balance.

4. Versatility in Workouts:

   - FIIT offers a diverse range of exercises, allowing for customization based on individual fitness levels and preferences. From bodyweight movements to incorporating equipment, FIIT provides a versatile platform that can be tailored to your weight loss journey.

5. HIIT Principles in FIIT:

   - FIIT incorporates High-Intensity Interval Training (HIIT) principles, maximizing cardiovascular benefits and fat burning. Understand how the strategic alternation between intense bursts of activity and rest periods amplifies the effectiveness of FIIT for weight loss.

6. Consistency and Long-Term Results:

   - Discover how the sustainable nature of FIIT makes it conducive to long-term weight loss success. By fostering a habit of consistent, challenging workouts, FIIT becomes a key ally in achieving and maintaining a healthy weight.

7. Nutritional Synergy with FIIT:

   - Learn how proper nutrition complements FIIT for optimal weight loss results. Explore pre and post-workout nutrition strategies that align with the demands of FIIT, supporting energy levels, recovery, and overall well-being.

As you embark on your FIIT journey for weight loss, this information provides a roadmap to navigate the principles, benefits, and application of Functional Intensity Interval Training. Unleash the potential of FIIT to not only shed excess weight but also to elevate your overall fitness and well-being.

Recommendation:

I won't try to reinvent the wheel; instead, I want to guide you to a resource that's tailor-made for women and can significantly accelerate your HIIT weight loss journey. Allow me to recommend a book that specifically caters to the unique needs and goals of women, offering insights, exercises, and programs designed to bring about effective and efficient results. This book is not just a fitness guide; it's a companion crafted to empower women on their path to achieving weight loss success through the proven and dynamic method of High-Intensity Interval Training (HIIT). Let's expedite your fitness journey together with this invaluable resource!

High-Intensity Interval Training for Women: Achieve Your Best Body with Quick and Powerful Workouts! https://amzn.to/46waPPD

Revitalize your fitness journey with High-Intensity Interval Training (HIIT), specifically designed to empower and inspire women on their path to wellness! Unleash the incredible benefits of HIIT, a dynamic method that torches fat, builds strength, and fits seamlessly into your busy lifestyle.

Why Choose High-Intensity Interval Training for Women?

Efficiency and Speed: HIIT delivers rapid results with short, impactful workouts. Say goodbye to lengthy exercise sessions and hello to quick, effective routines tailored to your busy schedule.

Anywhere, Anytime Workouts: Discover 60 versatile

exercises targeting major muscle groups, with a focus on the core and lower body – areas women often prioritize. These exercises require minimal equipment and can be done wherever you are.

Step-by-Step Guidance: Navigate your fitness journey with confidence using clear, step-by-step instructions accompanied by stunning visuals for every exercise. Feel empowered to master each movement and maximize your workout potential.

Customizable Programs: Choose from over 45 expertly crafted routines suitable for all fitness levels. Embark on four multi-day challenges, ranging from three to invigorating 28-day programs, ensuring you stay engaged and motivated.

Comprehensive Approach: Dive into essential topics such as understanding HIIT, pre- and post-workout stretching, goal setting, and nutrition. Arm yourself with the knowledge needed to kickstart your journey and maintain lasting success.

Embark on a transformative fitness adventure with High-Intensity Interval Training for Women. Uncover the strength, energy, and confidence you deserve in a way that aligns with your unique lifestyle. Elevate your workout experience, achieve your fitness goals, and embrace the powerful, time-efficient world of HIIT!

HIIT for Men:

Hiit: The 20-Minute Dream Body with High Intensity
Interval Training

The 80/20 Rule

In the context of High-Intensity Interval Training
(HIIT), the term "80/20" typically refers to the principle
of training intensity distribution. The 80/20 rule
suggests that an effective training program should
consist of approximately 80% low to moderate-intensity
exercise and 20% high-intensity exercise.

This principle is derived from the observation that the
majority of an individual's workouts, especially in
endurance training, should be performed at a moderate
intensity to build a strong aerobic base. The remaining
20% involves incorporating high-intensity intervals to
push the limits and stimulate adaptations that contribute
to improved performance and fitness.

In HIIT, the 80/20 rule underscores the importance of
balancing intense, challenging intervals (the 20%) with
less strenuous, recovery periods or steady-state cardio
(the 80%). This distribution aims to optimize the
benefits of both low and high-intensity training,
fostering overall cardiovascular health, endurance, and
performance improvements.

It's important to note that the 80/20 ratio is a guideline,

and individual preferences, fitness levels, and specific training goals may warrant adjustments. Additionally, the ratio may vary across different HIIT protocols and programs. As with any fitness principle, the key is to find a balance that aligns with personal needs and promotes long-term sustainability in one's workout routine.

In my Optimal Fitness series, I offer a caution about starting slow and building from there. For a person who is just starting to exercise, I suggest starting slow and working your way up. Don't overdo it. I know you want to look ripped tomorrow but it is going to take a bit longer than one day, one workout.

Using the 80/20 rule and the P.O.P. approach to working out for beginnings, let's use running as an example. Start out with something you can handle. In other words, don't exercise to the extent that you hurt yourself. If you inflict injury to your body, you will NOT workout for a while and in many cases that is enough to get some people to quite.

Let's consider a scenario where you plan to run for 5 minutes. During the initial 4 minutes, maintain a reasonable pace without pushing yourself too hard. Reserve the last minute for giving it your all. If you find it challenging to sprint for one minute, it's crucial to stop and avoid any risk of injury.

In the beginning, you might need to either decrease your total runtime or, if the first 4 minutes feel comfortable, wait until you can incorporate a high-intensity interval into the last 1 minute. Once you can successfully execute a five-minute run with the last minute in HIIT mode, you can gradually increase the overall running time.

By incrementally adding just 0.5 minutes to your run each week, within six months, you'll be running for nearly 20 minutes. Considering that twenty percent of 20 minutes is 4 minutes, you'll have achieved a significant progression.

It's worth noting that you don't have to run outdoors; you can achieve the same effect by simply running in place.

Fueling the Fire

The Crucial Role of Carbohydrates in HIIT Performance

Carbohydrates play a crucial role in High-Intensity Interval Training (HIIT) for several reasons, contributing to both energy production and overall performance. Here are the key reasons why carbohydrates are important in the context of HIIT:

1. Primary Energy Source:

   - Carbohydrates are the body's preferred and most efficient source of energy. During high-intensity exercises, such as those performed in HIIT, the body relies heavily on carbohydrates to fuel the intense bursts of activity. Having an adequate supply of carbohydrates ensures that your body has the energy needed to perform at its best during the high-intensity intervals.

2. Glycogen Storage:

   - Carbohydrates are stored in the muscles and liver as glycogen. These glycogen stores act as a readily available reservoir of energy that can be quickly mobilized during intense physical activity. HIIT often depletes glycogen stores, and having sufficient carbohydrates in your diet helps maintain these energy reserves for optimal performance.

3. Sustained Energy:

- HIIT workouts involve rapid transitions between high-intensity efforts and brief rest periods. Carbohydrates provide a quick and easily accessible source of energy, ensuring that you can maintain the intensity throughout the workout. Consuming carbohydrates before a HIIT session can help sustain energy levels and delay fatigue.

4. Improved Endurance:

- Carbohydrates contribute to endurance by providing a steady supply of glucose, which is the body's primary fuel for aerobic metabolism. This is particularly important in longer HIIT sessions or workouts with multiple intervals, where sustained energy is crucial for overall performance.

5. Enhanced Recovery:

- After a HIIT session, glycogen stores may be depleted, and the body requires carbohydrates to replenish these stores. Consuming carbohydrates post-workout, especially within the first 30 minutes to an hour, helps kickstart the recovery process by refueling glycogen stores and facilitating muscle repair.

6. Blood Sugar Regulation:

- Maintaining stable blood sugar levels is essential for sustained energy and overall well-being. Consuming carbohydrates in the right balance before a HIIT workout helps regulate blood sugar levels, preventing energy crashes during the session.

7. Minimizing Protein Usage for Energy:

- Carbohydrates spare protein from being used as an energy source. When carbohydrates are insufficient, the body may resort to breaking down muscle protein for energy. By ensuring an adequate carbohydrate intake, you can help preserve muscle mass and support muscle function during HIIT.

In summary, carbohydrates are a vital component of an effective HIIT nutrition strategy. Ensuring that you have an appropriate amount of carbohydrates in your diet, both before and after HIIT sessions, can optimize energy levels, enhance performance, and support the recovery process. Keep in mind that individual carbohydrate needs may vary based on factors such as fitness level, workout intensity, and overall dietary goals. Consulting with a nutrition professional can help tailor carbohydrate intake to meet your specific needs.

Powering Performance

The Vital Role of Protein in High-Intensity Interval Training (HIIT)

Embark on a comprehensive exploration into the cornerstone of High-Intensity Interval Training (HIIT) nutrition – protein. This chapter unravels the significance of protein in elevating your HIIT experience, providing a detailed understanding of why this macronutrient is indispensable for not only performance but also recovery, muscle preservation, and overall fitness excellence.

1. Muscle Support and Repair:

   - Synopsis: Dive into the foundational role of protein in supporting and repairing muscles, crucial for the demands placed on the body during intense HIIT sessions. Uncover the science behind protein's ability to aid in muscle recovery and minimize post-workout soreness.

2. Energy During Prolonged HIIT:

   - Synopsis: Explore how protein, while not the primary energy source, contributes to sustained energy during prolonged HIIT sessions. Understand its role in preventing muscle breakdown and ensuring a steady stream of amino acids for energy production.

3. Lean Muscle Mass Preservation:

- Synopsis: Delve into the unique aspect of protein as a guardian of lean muscle mass. Learn how protein intake can counteract the potential loss of muscle mass that may occur during extended HIIT training periods, contributing to a sculpted and defined physique.

4. Appetite Regulation:

- Synopsis: Uncover the satiating power of protein and its impact on appetite regulation. Explore how including an adequate amount of protein in your HIIT nutrition plan can assist in managing cravings, promoting a healthy relationship with food.

5. Post-Workout Recovery:

- Synopsis: Peer into the post-HIIT recovery landscape and understand how protein aids in the repair and rebuilding of muscle tissue. Gain insights into the optimal timing and composition of post-workout protein intake for maximizing recovery benefits.

6. Amino Acid Profile:

- Synopsis: Explore the diverse world of amino acids, the building blocks of protein. Understand the importance of a balanced amino acid profile in supporting various physiological functions, from immune system function to neurotransmitter synthesis.

7. Hydration and Protein Utilization:

- Synopsis: Uncover the synergistic relationship between hydration and protein utilization. Learn how staying adequately hydrated enhances the body's ability to absorb and utilize protein effectively, optimizing its benefits for HIIT enthusiasts.

8. Individualized Protein Needs:

- Synopsis: Recognize the variability in protein requirements among individuals based on factors such as age, gender, activity level, and fitness goals. Gain insights into tailoring your protein intake to meet your specific needs for optimal HIIT performance.

In summary, this chapter serves as a comprehensive guide to the pivotal role of protein in powering your HIIT journey. From muscle support and recovery to lean muscle preservation and appetite regulation, protein emerges as an indispensable ally in the quest for fitness excellence. Tailor your protein intake to align with your unique needs and goals, ensuring that this macronutrient serves as a cornerstone for your optimal performance in the dynamic world of High-Intensity Interval Training.

Aggie

One of the people I follow in Instagram is Aggie. She borrowed $10K from her Dad to attend a Tony Robbins seminar and gained fame in making her first $1,000,000 nine months later. She has inspired thousands of people with her Biohacking coaching.

Aggie recommends for people wanting to lose weight to eat meals in the following order:

- Fibers

- Proteins and Fats

- Carbohydrates

- Sweet and Treats

In my book, "Biohacking Blueprint: A Journey to Personal Transformation", I go into more detail about how to use Aggie's advise for daily food consumption. A example of a typical meal plan for one day based on the Fiber-Proteins/Fats-Carb-Sweets scheme is:

Breakfast: Fiber-Rich Smoothie Bowl

- Greek yogurt base

- Mixed berries (raspberries, blueberries)

- Chia seeds

- Flaxseeds

- Topped with sliced almonds

Mid-Morning Snack: Protein and Fat-Packed Snack

- Hard-boiled eggs

- Avocado slices

- Sprinkle of sea salt

Lunch: Quinoa Salad with Grilled Chicken

- Quinoa

- Grilled chicken breast

- Mixed veggies (cucumbers, cherry tomatoes, bell peppers)

- Olive oil and lemon dressing

Afternoon Snack: Carb and Protein Combo

- Whole grain rice cakes

- Hummus

- Cherry tomatoes

Dinner: Sweet Potato and Chickpea Curry

- Sweet potato and chickpea curry

- Basmati rice

- Side of steamed broccoli

Evening Snack: Sweet and Nutty Treat

- Greek yogurt

- Drizzle of honey

- Mixed nuts (almonds, walnuts)

Hydration:

- Water or herbal tea throughout the day

Dessert: Dark Chocolate and Berries

- Dark chocolate squares

- Mixed berries (strawberries, blackberries)

Here is another:

Breakfast:

- 1 cup steel-cut oatmeal with mixed berries (Fiber)

- 2 eggs or a protein-rich plant-based alternative such as tofu scramble (Proteins/Fats)

- 1 slice of whole-wheat bread, dry or with a light spread of avocado (Carb)

Mid-Morning Snack:

- 1 oz almonds or walnuts (Proteins/Fats)

- Apple or a pear (Fiber)

Lunch:

- Large spinach salad with cucumber, tomato, avocado, and grilled chicken breast or chickpeas (Proteins/Fats & Fiber)

- 1/2 cup brown rice or quinoa (Carb)

Afternoon Snack:

- Baby carrots or cut bell peppers dipped in hummus (Fiber & Proteins/Fats)

Dinner:

- Grilled salmon fillet or lentil stew (Proteins/Fats)

- Steamed broccoli and cauliflower (Fiber)

- Sweet potato, baked or mashed (Carb)

Dessert/Sweet treat (optional):

- A square of dark chocolate with a minimum of 70% cocoa content, preferably sugar-free or low in refined sugar. Alternatively, have a small portion of fresh fruit if you prefer natural sweets.

Note:

- This meal plan is a general guideline and can be adjusted based on individual dietary preferences and caloric needs.

- Prioritize whole, nutrient-dense foods to support overall health and fitness goals.

- Adjust portion sizes based on your individual requirements and goals.

- Ensure proper hydration, especially around your HIIT workout sessions.

This meal plan emphasizes a balance of fiber-rich foods, lean proteins, and healthy fats, followed by complex carbohydrates and a small dessert. Remember to customize the plan according to your nutritional needs, preferences, and fitness goals. If you have specific dietary concerns, consider consulting with a registered dietitian or nutrition professional for personalized advice.

For more detailed information about Fibers-Proteins/Fats-Carbs-Sweets see:

https://amzn.to/3RdRvlW

The Benefits of Embracing Beans

A Gateway to Weight Loss and Gut Health

From my book, *"Easy-Peasy Weight Loss: Simplifying Your Journey to a Healthier You"*, I am including this excerpt about *"7 Foods That Aid in Burning Belly Fat."*

Beyond being a rich source of soluble fiber, beans play a pivotal role in reducing inflammation in the digestive system. Chronic inflammation, a potential consequence of dietary choices, can contribute to weight gain. By incorporating beans into your meals, not only do you introduce a weight-loss-friendly food, but you also promote gut health and address inflammation issues.

Strategic Fat Inclusion:

Swapping Beef for Salmon

Contrary to popular belief, eliminating fats entirely from your diet is not a sustainable or healthy approach to weight loss. The key lies in making informed choices about the types of fats you consume. Saturated fats from meat and dairy can hinder weight loss goals, but opting for polyunsaturated fats, such as those found in salmon, is a more beneficial strategy. While salmon alone may not directly cause weight loss, making this dietary swap is a step in the right direction, as highlighted by insights from San Francisco Gate.

Yogurt's Weight-Loss Superpower:

A Triple Threat Against Fat

Research reveals that integrating three servings of fat-free yogurt into a reduced-calorie diet significantly enhances fat and weight loss. Compared to those on a similar calorie-restricted diet without yogurt, individuals consuming yogurt lost 22% more weight and an impressive 61% more body fat. This yogurt-induced fat-burning effect showcases the potential of this dairy product as a valuable ally in weight loss efforts.

Red Bell Peppers:

A Vitamin C Boost for Belly Fat Combat

Packed with three times the recommended daily intake of vitamin C, red bell peppers emerge as a potent weapon against belly fat. The vitamin C content, comparable to that found in citrus fruits, can be a crucial element in your arsenal against weight gain. Including these vibrant vegetables in your diet becomes a flavorful and nutritious strategy for achieving your weight loss goals.

Broccoli and Hummus:

A Dynamic Duo for Nutrient-Rich Meals

High in vitamin C, broccoli proves to be a nutritional

powerhouse. When paired with hummus, this combination not only enhances the flavor of your meal but also provides a satisfying and nutrient-rich option. Embracing this duo offers a delicious way to incorporate essential vitamins into your diet while contributing to your weight loss journey.

Edamame:

Fiber-Rich Satiety with Low Caloric Impact

Acting as an ideal side dish, edamame brings a double benefit to the table – high fiber and nutrient content coupled with remarkably low calories. This combination makes edamame an excellent choice for those aiming to feel full for an extended period while managing their caloric intake. Including edamame in your meals can be a strategic move in your weight loss plan.

Diluted Vinegar:

Unveiling the Potential of Acetic Acid for Metabolism Boost

The trendy health food, apple cider vinegar, might hold more benefits than meets the eye. According to Professor Carol Johnston from Arizona State University, acetic acid in vinegar could potentially activate fat metabolism. While more research is needed, preliminary findings suggest that diluted vinegar, when consumed responsibly, might boost metabolism. Johnston advises against consuming vinegar undiluted, emphasizing potential health risks, and recommends a diluted solution of two tablespoons of vinegar with 8 ounces of water for a safer and potentially beneficial experience.

HIIT Carbohydrate Meals

Here are HIIT-friendly recipes with a focus on incorporating carbohydrates:

1. Quinoa and Veggie Power Bowl:

- Ingredients:

  - 1 cup cooked quinoa

  - 1 cup mixed vegetables (broccoli, bell peppers, carrots)

  - 1/2 cup chickpeas (canned, drained, and rinsed)

  - 1 tablespoon olive oil

  - 1 teaspoon lemon juice

  - Salt and pepper to taste

- Instructions:

   1. Sauté mixed vegetables in olive oil until tender.

   2. Mix cooked quinoa, chickpeas, and sautéed vegetables in a bowl.

   3. Drizzle with lemon juice, season with salt and pepper, and toss.

2. Sweet Potato and Black Bean Burrito Bowl:

- Ingredients:

  - 1 cup cooked brown rice

  - 1 sweet potato, diced and roasted

  - 1/2 cup black beans (canned, drained, and rinsed)

- Salsa and guacamole for topping

- Fresh cilantro for garnish

- Instructions:

1. Assemble a bowl with brown rice, roasted sweet potatoes, and black beans.

2. Top with salsa, guacamole, and fresh cilantro.

3. Whole Grain Pasta with Pesto and Cherry Tomatoes:

- Ingredients:

    - 1 cup whole grain pasta, cooked

    - 2 tablespoons pesto sauce

    - 1 cup cherry tomatoes, halved

    - 1/4 cup grated Parmesan cheese

    - Fresh basil for garnish

- Instructions:

    1. Toss cooked pasta with pesto sauce.

    2. Mix in cherry tomatoes and top with Parmesan cheese.

    3. Garnish with fresh basil.

4. Brown Rice Stir-Fry with Tofu and Vegetables:

- Ingredients:

  - 1 cup cooked brown rice

  - 1/2 cup extra-firm tofu, cubed

  - 1 cup mixed stir-fry vegetables (broccoli, snap peas, carrots)

  - 2 tablespoons soy sauce

  - 1 tablespoon sesame oil

- Instructions:

  1. Sauté tofu until golden brown.

  2. Add mixed vegetables and stir-fry until tender.

  3. Mix in cooked brown rice, soy sauce, and sesame oil.

5. Mango and Black Bean Quinoa Salad:

- Ingredients:

  - 1 cup cooked quinoa

  - 1 mango, diced

  - 1/2 cup black beans (canned, drained, and rinsed)

  - 1/4 cup red onion, finely chopped

  - Fresh lime juice for dressing

- Instructions:

  1. Combine cooked quinoa, diced mango, black beans, and red onion in a bowl.

  2. Drizzle with fresh lime juice and toss gently.

6. Chickpea and Spinach Stuffed Sweet Potatoes:

  - Ingredients:

    - 2 medium-sized sweet potatoes

    - 1 can chickpeas, drained and rinsed

    - 2 cups fresh spinach, chopped

    - 1 tablespoon olive oil

    - 1 teaspoon cumin

    - Salt and pepper to taste

  - Instructions:

    1. Bake sweet potatoes until tender.

    2. Sauté chickpeas and spinach in olive oil with cumin, salt, and pepper.

    3. Cut sweet potatoes in half, scoop out a bit of flesh, and fill with the chickpea-spinach mixture.

7. Brown Rice and Lentil Bowl with Roasted Veggies:

   - Ingredients:

     - 1 cup cooked brown rice

     - 1/2 cup dry lentils, cooked

     - Assorted roasted vegetables (zucchini, cherry tomatoes, bell peppers)

     - 2 tablespoons balsamic vinaigrette

     - Fresh herbs for garnish

   - Instructions:

     1. Combine cooked brown rice and lentils in a bowl.

     2. Top with roasted vegetables and drizzle with balsamic vinaigrette.

     3. Garnish with fresh herbs.

8. Quinoa and Berry Parfait:

- Ingredients:

  - 1 cup cooked quinoa

  - Mixed berries (strawberries, blueberries, raspberries)

  - 1/2 cup Greek yogurt

  - 1 tablespoon honey

  - Chopped nuts for crunch

- Instructions:

  1. Layer cooked quinoa, mixed berries, and Greek yogurt in a glass or bowl.

  2. Drizzle with honey and top with chopped nuts.

9. Spaghetti Squash Primavera:

- Ingredients:

  - 1 medium-sized spaghetti squash

  - Assorted sautéed vegetables (zucchini, cherry tomatoes, mushrooms)

  - 2 tablespoons olive oil

  - Garlic, herbs, and Parmesan for seasoning

- Instructions:

  1. Roast spaghetti squash until strands are easily fluffed with a fork.

  2. Sauté vegetables in olive oil, season with garlic, herbs, and Parmesan.

  3. Toss vegetables with spaghetti squash strands.

10. Couscous and Chickpea Salad:

- Ingredients:

    - 1 cup cooked couscous

    - 1 can chickpeas, drained and rinsed

    - Diced cucumber, cherry tomatoes, and red onion

    - Lemon-tahini dressing

    - Fresh parsley for garnish

- Instructions:

    1. Combine cooked couscous, chickpeas, and diced vegetables in a bowl.

    2. Drizzle with lemon-tahini dressing and toss.

    3. Garnish with fresh parsley.

These recipes provide a variety of flavors and nutrients to support your energy needs during HIIT workouts. They also offer a balance of carbohydrates, protein, and healthy fats to fuel your HIIT workouts effectively. Adjust portion sizes based on your nutritional needs and fitness goals.

HIIT Protein Meals

Here are ten HIIT-friendly meals with a focus on protein, along with ingredients and instructions:

1. Grilled Chicken and Quinoa Salad:

- Ingredients:
    - Grilled chicken breast
    - 1 cup cooked quinoa
    - Mixed greens
    - Cherry tomatoes, cucumber, and red onion
    - Balsamic vinaigrette

- Instructions:
    1. Grill chicken breast and slice.
    2. Combine quinoa, mixed greens, sliced chicken, and chopped vegetables.
    3. Drizzle with balsamic vinaigrette and toss.

2. Salmon and Asparagus Foil Packets:

- Ingredients:
    - Salmon fillets
    - Asparagus spears
    - Lemon slices

- Olive oil, garlic, and herbs

- Salt and pepper

- Instructions:

1. Place salmon fillets and asparagus on a foil sheet.

2. Drizzle with olive oil, add garlic, herbs, and lemon slices.

3. Seal the foil and bake until salmon is cooked through.

3. Turkey and Sweet Potato Skillet:

- Ingredients:

- Ground turkey

- Sweet potatoes, diced

- Bell peppers, onions, and spinach

- Taco seasoning

- Avocado for topping

- Instructions:

1. Brown ground turkey in a skillet.

2. Add diced sweet potatoes and sauté until tender.

3. Mix in bell peppers, onions, and spinach, and season with taco seasoning.

4. Top with sliced avocado.

4. Egg White Omelette with Spinach and Feta:

- Ingredients:

    - Egg whites

    - Fresh spinach

    - Feta cheese

    - Cherry tomatoes, diced

    - Olive oil

- Instructions:

    1. Whisk egg whites and pour into a heated pan.

    2. Add spinach, feta, and diced tomatoes.

    3. Fold the omelette and cook until set.

5. Lean Beef and Broccoli Stir-Fry:

- Ingredients:

    - Lean beef strips

    - Broccoli florets

    - Soy sauce, ginger, and garlic

    - Brown rice

    - Sesame seeds for garnish

- Instructions:

    1. Stir-fry beef strips until browned.

    2. Add broccoli and sauté with soy sauce, ginger, and

garlic.

3. Serve over cooked brown rice and garnish with sesame seeds.

6. Chickpea and Spinach Curry:

- Ingredients:

- Chickpeas (canned, drained, and rinsed)

- Fresh spinach

- Coconut milk

- Curry spices (turmeric, cumin, coriander)

- Basmati rice

- Instructions:

1. Simmer chickpeas, spinach, and coconut milk with curry spices.

2. Serve over cooked basmati rice.

7. Shrimp and Avocado Wrap:

- Ingredients:

  - Grilled shrimp

  - Whole wheat wrap

  - Avocado slices

  - Lettuce and cherry tomatoes

  - Greek yogurt sauce

- Instructions:

  1. Fill a whole wheat wrap with grilled shrimp, avocado, lettuce, and tomatoes.

  2. Drizzle with Greek yogurt sauce.

  3.

8. Tofu and Vegetable Skewers:

- Ingredients:

  - Firm tofu cubes

  - Bell peppers, zucchini, and cherry tomatoes

  - Olive oil and balsamic glaze

  - Quinoa for serving

- Instructions:

  1. Skewer tofu cubes and vegetables.

  2. Grill or bake, drizzle with olive oil and balsamic glaze.

  3. Serve over quinoa.

9. Lentil and Kale Soup:

  - Ingredients:

   - Brown lentils

   - Kale leaves, chopped

   - Carrots, celery, and onions

   - Vegetable broth

   - Cumin and paprika for seasoning

  - Instructions:

   1. Simmer lentils, kale, vegetables, and broth with cumin and paprika.

   2. Cook until lentils are tender.

10. Greek Yogurt Parfait with Berries and Nuts:

  - Ingredients:

   - Greek yogurt

   - Mixed berries (strawberries, blueberries, raspberries)

   - Almonds or walnuts

   - Honey for drizzling

  - Instructions:

   1. Layer Greek yogurt with mixed berries in a glass.

   2. Top with nuts and drizzle with honey.

These protein-packed meals offer a variety of flavors and nutrients to support your energy needs during HIIT workouts. Adjust portion sizes based on your individual requirements.

HIIT Fats Meals

Here are ten HIIT-friendly meals with a focus on healthy fats, along with ingredients and instructions:

1. Avocado and Grilled Chicken Salad:

 - Ingredients:

   - Grilled chicken breast

   - Mixed greens

   - Cherry tomatoes, cucumber, and red onion

   - Avocado slices

   - Olive oil and balsamic vinaigrette

 - Instructions:

   1. Grill chicken breast and slice.

   2. Combine mixed greens, cherry tomatoes, cucumber, red onion, and avocado slices.

   3. Drizzle with a mix of olive oil and balsamic vinaigrette.

2. Salmon and Quinoa Stuffed Peppers:

- Ingredients:

    - Salmon fillets

    - Quinoa, cooked

    - Bell peppers, halved

    - Spinach and feta cheese

    - Lemon and herbs

- Instructions:

    1. Bake salmon fillets and flake into cooked quinoa.

    2. Mix with spinach, feta, and herbs.

    3. Stuff bell peppers and bake until tender.

3. Walnut-Crusted Tilapia with Roasted Vegetables:

- Ingredients:

  - Tilapia fillets

  - Crushed walnuts

  - Asparagus, carrots, and Brussels sprouts

  - Olive oil, garlic, and lemon

- Instructions:

  1. Coat tilapia in crushed walnuts and bake.

  2. Roast vegetables with olive oil, garlic, and lemon.

4. Mediterranean Chickpea Salad:

- Ingredients:

  - Chickpeas (canned, drained, and rinsed)

  - Cucumber, cherry tomatoes, and red onion

  - Feta cheese and Kalamata olives

  - Olive oil and lemon juice

- Instructions:

  1. Combine chickpeas, cucumber, tomatoes, red onion, feta, and olives.

  2. Drizzle with olive oil and lemon juice.

5. Coconut-Curry Chicken Skewers:

- Ingredients:

  - Chicken skewers

  - Coconut milk and curry paste

  - Bell peppers and red onion

  - Coconut flakes for garnish

- Instructions:

  1. Marinate chicken in coconut milk and curry paste.

  2. Skewer with bell peppers and red onion.

  3. Grill and garnish with coconut flakes.

6. Tuna and Avocado Lettuce Wraps:

- Ingredients:

  - Canned tuna, drained

  - Avocado, mashed

  - Lettuce leaves

  - Cherry tomatoes and cucumber

  - Olive oil and lemon

- Instructions:

  1. Mix tuna with mashed avocado.

  2. Spoon into lettuce leaves and top with tomatoes and cucumber.

  3. Drizzle with olive oil and lemon.

7. Spaghetti Squash with Pesto and Pine Nuts:

- Ingredients:

  - Roasted spaghetti squash

  - Basil pesto

  - Cherry tomatoes and spinach

  - Toasted pine nuts

- Instructions:

  1. Toss roasted spaghetti squash with pesto.

2. Mix in cherry tomatoes, spinach, and top with pine nuts.

8. Almond-Crusted Chicken Tenders:

- Ingredients:

  - Chicken tenders

  - Almond flour and paprika

  - Eggs for dipping

  - Broccoli and cauliflower florets

- Instructions:

1. Coat chicken tenders in a mix of almond flour and paprika.

2. Dip in beaten eggs and bake.

3. Serve with roasted broccoli and cauliflower.

9. Greek Yogurt and Berry Smoothie Bowl:

- Ingredients:

  - Greek yogurt

  - Mixed berries (strawberries, blueberries, raspberries)

  - Chia seeds and shredded coconut

- Instructions:

  1. Blend Greek yogurt and berries into a smoothie.

  2. Pour into a bowl and top with chia seeds and shredded coconut.

10. Olive and Tomato Quinoa Stuffed Bell Peppers:

- Ingredients:

  - Quinoa, cooked

  - Black olives, sliced

  - Cherry tomatoes, diced

  - Feta cheese

  - Bell peppers, halved

- Instructions:

  1. Mix cooked quinoa with olives, tomatoes, and feta.

  2. Stuff bell peppers and bake until tender.

These meals provide a balance of healthy fats to support your energy needs during HIIT workouts. Adjust portion sizes based on your individual requirements.

HIIT Friendly Sweets and Desserts

Here are ten HIIT-friendly sweets and desserts with a focus on balance and nutrition, along with ingredients and instructions:

1. Protein-Packed Chocolate Smoothie Bowl:

- Ingredients:

  - Chocolate protein powder

  - Frozen banana

  - Almond milk

  - Toppings: Chopped nuts, shredded coconut, and dark chocolate chips

- Instructions:

  1. Blend chocolate protein powder, frozen banana, and almond milk until smooth.

  2. Pour into a bowl and top with chopped nuts, shredded coconut, and dark chocolate chips.

2. Greek Yogurt Parfait:

- Ingredients:

  - Greek yogurt

  - Mixed berries (blueberries, strawberries)

- Granola

- Honey for drizzling

- Instructions:

1. Layer Greek yogurt, mixed berries, and granola in a glass.

2. Drizzle with honey.

3. Chia Seed Pudding with Mango:

- Ingredients:

- Chia seeds

- Almond milk

- Mango, diced

- Vanilla extract

- Instructions:

1. Mix chia seeds, almond milk, and vanilla extract in a jar.

2. Refrigerate overnight.

3. Top with diced mango before serving.

4. Baked Apple with Cinnamon:

- Ingredients:

- Apple, cored and sliced

- Cinnamon

- Greek yogurt

- Instructions:

1. Sprinkle apple slices with cinnamon.

2. Bake until tender.

3. Serve with a dollop of Greek yogurt.

5. Coconut and Berry Nice Cream:

- Ingredients:

- Frozen mixed berries

- Coconut milk

- Shredded coconut

- Instructions:

1. Blend frozen berries and coconut milk until creamy.

2. Top with shredded coconut.

6. Dark Chocolate-Dipped Strawberries:

- Ingredients:

- Dark chocolate (70% cocoa or higher)

- Fresh strawberries

  - Instructions:

    1. Melt dark chocolate.

    2. Dip strawberries into melted chocolate.

    3. Place on parchment paper to cool.

7. Almond Butter and Banana Bites:

  - Ingredients:

    - Sliced bananas

    - Almond butter

    - Chopped almonds

  - Instructions:

    1. Spread almond butter on banana slices.

    2. Sprinkle with chopped almonds.

8. Oatmeal Raisin Energy Balls:

- Ingredients:

  - Rolled oats

  - Raisins

  - Almond butter

  - Honey

- Instructions:

  1. Mix rolled oats, raisins, almond butter, and honey.

  2. Form into small balls and refrigerate.

9. Peach and Yogurt Popsicles:

- Ingredients:

  - Fresh or frozen peaches

  - Greek yogurt

  - Honey

- Instructions:

  1. Blend peaches, Greek yogurt, and honey.

  2. Pour into popsicle molds and freeze.

10. Cocoa-Dusted Almonds:

- Ingredients:

    - Raw almonds

    - Cocoa powder

    - Stevia or sweetener of choice

- Instructions:

    1. Toss raw almonds in cocoa powder and sweetener.

    2. Roast until crisp.

These sweets and desserts are designed to provide a satisfying treat while incorporating nutritious ingredients. Adjust portion sizes based on your dietary preferences and fitness goals.

In Summary

High-Intensity Interval Training (HIIT) offers a multitude of benefits, making it a dynamic and efficient approach to achieving optimal fitness goals. These advantages include enhanced cardiovascular health, increased metabolic rate, fat loss, improved oxygen consumption, and muscle preservation. The uniqueness of HIIT lies in its time efficiency and adaptability to various fitness levels and goals.

Consistency and persistence are pivotal in realizing the full potential of HIIT. Regular engagement ensures the body continually adapts to the intensity, resulting in sustained improvements. As with any fitness journey, patience is key. The transformative effects of HIIT often unfold gradually, and persistence through challenges is crucial.

A successful HIIT journey involves understanding individual fitness levels, setting realistic goals, and embracing the adaptability of HIIT workouts. Tailoring routines to personal preferences and gradually progressing in intensity fosters a sustainable commitment. Safety considerations, such as proper warm-up and consulting healthcare professionals, are paramount, especially for beginners.

Motivation is the driving force behind success in HIIT. Celebrate small victories, track progress, and find joy in the process. The journey to optimal fitness is unique for each individual, and embracing this uniqueness fosters a positive mindset. Surrounding oneself with a supportive community or seeking guidance from fitness professionals can provide encouragement during challenging moments.

In essence, HIIT's transformative power is not solely in its scientific principles but in the consistent and persistent commitment to the journey. The path to optimal fitness is marked by gradual progress, a resilient mindset, and a celebration of every step taken toward a healthier, stronger self. By embracing the journey with dedication and positivity, individuals can unlock the full potential of HIIT and achieve their optimal fitness goals.

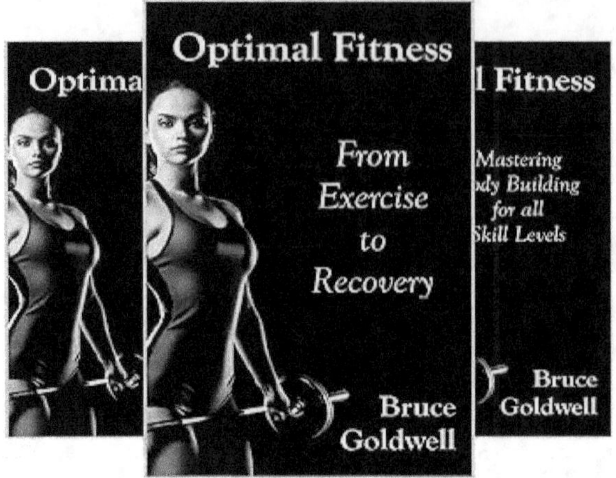

https://amzn.to/47wZe3E

Optimal Fitness: Pathways to a Healthier, More Robust You

"Discover the Secrets to a Longer, Healthier Life

with this Comprehensive Collection of Lifestyle Transformation Books!

In this curated selection of empowering reads, you'll find a wealth of knowledge and guidance on how to rejuvenate your life and embrace a healthier, longer, and more vibrant future. These books offer a holistic approach to well-being, covering everything from nutrition and fitness to stress management and mental resilience.

Learn how to make mindful dietary choices that nourish your body, explore invigorating exercise routines, and tap into stress-reduction techniques that promote mental and emotional equilibrium. Dive into the science of longevity, uncovering the latest research on habits that can extend your lifespan while enhancing your quality of life.

Our collection of books is designed to inspire and motivate you to take proactive steps toward a healthier, more fulfilling existence. Whether you're embarking on a new wellness journey or seeking to refine your current lifestyle, these resources will empower you with the tools and knowledge needed to craft a brighter and longer future.

Join the countless individuals who have embraced these insights and made positive changes in their lives. Start your transformative journey today and embrace the potential for a life of vitality, happiness, and longevity."

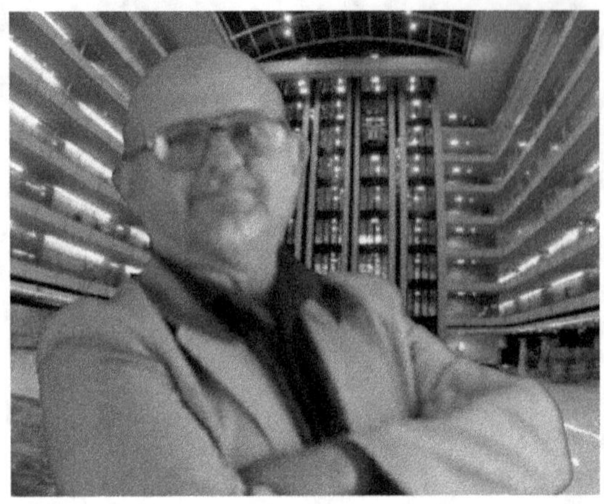

About The Author

Bruce Goldwell is a self-help/motivational author and creator of two captivating fantasy adventures, "Dragon Keepers" a six book series and "Starfighters Defending Earth" a three book series. He is an inspiring figure who has overcome significant challenges in his life. As a Vietnam veteran, he experienced homelessness for over ten years. During these difficult times, Bruce developed a compassionate heart and strong desire to uplift others. While living on the streets, he immersed himself in motivational literature at local bookstores, where he found solace in the works of renowned authors such as the creators of Chicken Soup for the Soul, Bob Proctor, and David Stanley, Elvis Presley's brother.

Inspired by the transformative impact of the film "The Secret," Goldwell penned his first book, "Mastery of Abundant Living: The Keys to Mastering the Law of Attraction." He had the honor of personally presenting the first autographed copy to Bob Proctor. Recognizing that young readers may not typically engage with self-help material, Goldwell brilliantly crafted a fantastical adventure series for teens. Within these enchanting stories, he weaves principles of success and powerful life lessons to ignite hope and encourage personal growth in younger audiences.

Driven by an unwavering belief in the power of his books to change lives, Bruce Goldwell's moving journey from homeless veteran to impactful author has resonated with thousands around the globe. His triumphant quest to help others is a testament to resilience, determination, and the transformative power of words.

Www.mykindlebooks.net